How You Were Born

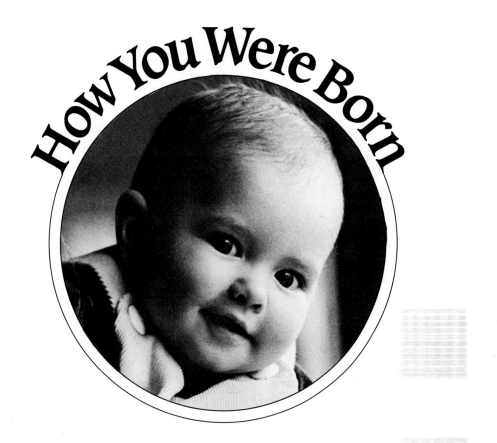

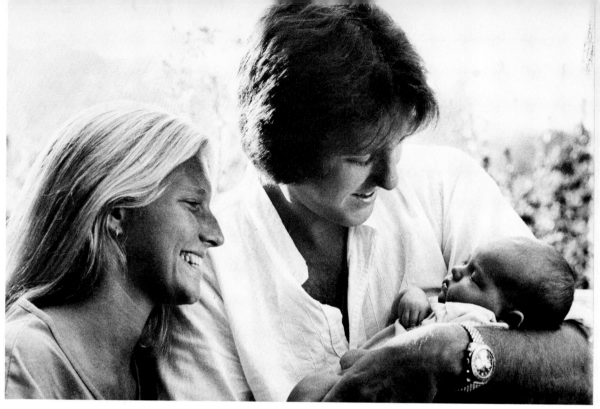

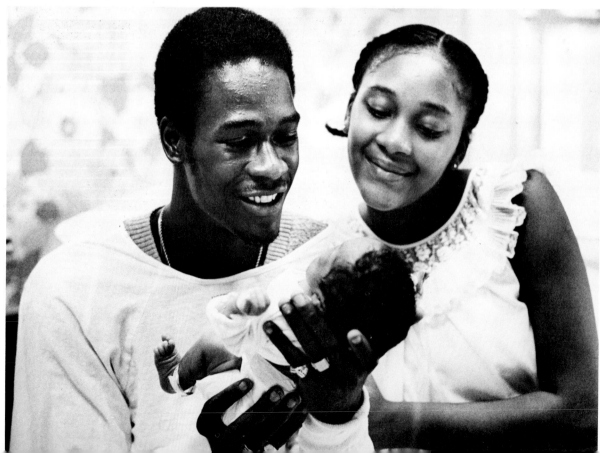

How You Were Born

BY
JOANNA COLE

William Morrow & Company
New York • 1984

ACKNOWLEDGEMENTS
The author wishes to thank Louise Bates Ames,
Anne C. Bernstein, and Dr. David Kliot for reading and
suggesting changes in the manuscript for this book.

PHOTO CREDITS: Susan Cole: p. 5; Tim Davis/Photo Researchers: p. 46 (top right); Richard Frieman/Photo Researchers: p. 44; Vivienne della Grotta/Photo Researchers: p. 46 (bottom); Hella Hammid: pp. 1, 2 (both), 24, 26, 27, 28, 32, 33, 34, 37, 39 (both), 43, 45 (top), 48; Barbara Kirk: p. 46 (top left); David Krasnor/Photo Researchers: p. 41; Inger McCabe/Photo Researchers: p. 36; Margaret Miller: p. 47; Lennart Nilsson (from *A Child Is Born*): pp. 10, 13, 20, 22; Thomas Stalling/Photo Researchers: p. 45 (bottom); Suzanne Szasz/Photo Researchers: pp. 15, 40, 42; Drawings by Ray Burns.

Printed in the United States of America.

10 9 8 7 6 5 4 3 2 1

Library of Congress Cataloging in Publication Data
Cole, Joanna.   How you were born.
Bibliography: p. Summary: Text and photos explain how a baby is conceived, how it grows inside the mother's womb, and how it is born.
1. Pregnancy—Juvenile literature. 2. Childbirth—Juvenile literature. [1. Pregnancy. 2. Childbirth. 3. Babies] I. Title.
RG525.5.C64   1984   612'.63   83-17314
ISBN 0-688-1710-X
ISBN 0-688-1709-6 (lib. bdg.)

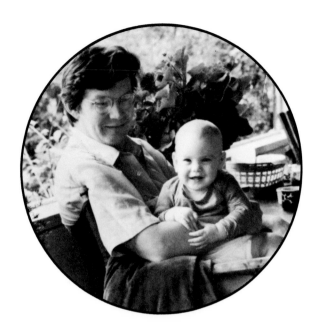

For Rachel

A Note to Parents

It is natural for children to ask "Why?" Just as they are curious about how a telephone works or what snow is made of, children also wonder where they came from and how they were born. When their questions are answered in a natural, open way, they can feel good about themselves and their feelings, trusting in the adults in their life.

So one good reason for talking with children about birth is that it shows them that you approve of them and their natural curiosity, and it helps them feel secure. But there is another reason as well, and that is to clear up confusion. Misunderstandings about birth and reproduction are common among children. For instance, having heard that a baby grows in its mother's "tummy," children sometimes worry that the infant is being showered with chunks of pizza or hot coffee. The notion of sperm as "seed" engenders many horticultural images. Children may believe that they were planted in the ground or that a woman becomes pregnant by swallowing a seed. The idea of the ovum as an egg leads some children to think that they hatched from a chicken's egg or that they once were a baby bird. Some other common misconceptions are that babies are purchased at a store or hospital; that babies are born from the mother's navel, ureter, or anus; and that babies are manufactured, the way a doll might be constructed in a factory.

Ideas like these might seem harmless enough, even charming at first. But for some children they can cause disturbing worries, and a calm explanation of the facts can be reassuring. Because it is not always easy for an adult to predict what inaccurate ideas a child may have, it can help to answer children's questions first with one of your own: "What do you think?" Once you find out what a child is really asking, you'll be

6

in a better position to give a helpful answer based on the facts.

At a young age it may be difficult for children to grasp some concepts, no matter how well or how often they are explained. There is no need to worry about this. Children's view of the world and their capacity to understand keep expanding as they mature, and they need to ask the same questions over again, fitting the information into their new level of understanding.

The biological facts of how babies are born, however, cannot be separated from a child's feelings. A child is interested in hearing the story of her own birth—when it is told in a loving way—because it affirms her parents' love and her own sense of how much she has grown. Therefore, it is not necessary or desirable to assume a grave or instructional tone. The atmosphere parents wish to create when talking with children about birth and reproduction is a warm, honest, and reassuring one that tells children they are free to ask questions as often as they need to, and you will answer them as lovingly as you know how.

This book was designed to tell children the story of birth in a simple yet informative way. When I read it with my own child, I stop often to answer questions, talk about the pictures, and compare her own birth with what is described in the book.

Preschool children often have a consuming interest in babies and birth, but may not be ready for a straight reading of the text. A partial reading may be just as valuable. You can concentrate on reading that portion of the text that is most interesting to the child and just talk about what he sees in the pictures for the rest of the book. As a child grows, she may come back to the book ready and curious to find out more.

The information on cesarean birth was included because so many babies are born this way today. Children need to know that it is simply another way to be born, and that the important parts of birth—the happy expectation of parents and the warmth of the feelings between parents and baby—are the same.

A good time to reminisce about how a child was born is when a new baby is expected. Then a child likes to remember a time when he was the center of attention. Sharing memories about his own birth shows him that he is special to you and can't be displaced in your affections.

As parents and children read together, questions will come up. Many will be easy to answer, but some will not. Sometimes parents feel inadequate when they don't know all the answers. But reproduction is a complicated business, and no one can know everything about anything. The simplest way to handle your own ignorance is to admit it freely, saying "I don't know" or "I'm not sure." If it seems important to answer a question, you can try to find out by consulting other sources. At the end of this section are listed some books for parents that I have found helpful for getting more information and also in deciding how to word explanations and how much or how little to say to children at various ages.

The youngest children are usually not very interested in knowing how the sperm and ovum get together. But as they grow, they may wonder about this. When children ask, it is best to give simple, straightforward answers and to give only as much information as a child seems to want at the time. The books listed here will be especially helpful with this.

Some parents say that their children do not ask any questions and are not curious. Probably the children have as much natural curiosity as any, but they may have gotten the impression that birth and reproduction are not something to be talked about. If you would like to offer a child the opportunity to ask, you can open things up by saying something like, "Most children have questions about how babies are born. If you have any, I'm available to talk about them."

8

When parents establish this kind of open, caring relationship from an early age, children will have a reliable source of information and guidance to turn to as they grow. My hope is that this book can be a part of that relationship for you and your child.

Joanna Cole

FOR FURTHER READING:

A Child Is Born: The Drama of Life Before Birth. Photographs by Lennart Nilsson. Text by Axel Ingelman-Sundberg and Claes Wirsen. New York: Dell Publishing Co., Inc., 1969. A classic photographic study of the development of a baby in the womb and its birth.

The First Nine Months of Life by Geraldine Lux Flanagan. New York: Simon and Schuster, 1962. A sensitive description of prenatal development, illustrated with photographs and drawings.

The Flight of the Stork by Anne C. Bernstein, Ph.D. New York: Dell Publishing Co., Inc., 1980. A child psychologist explains how children understand birth at various ages and advises parents on how to tell children about birth and reproduction.

How Was I Born? A Photographic Story of Reproduction and Birth for Children by Lennart Nilsson. New York: Delacorte Press, 1975. A book intended for school-age children and young people, this contains much information on birth that will also be useful to parents.

Talking With Your Child About Sex by Arlene S. Uslander and Caroline Weiss, in consultation with Lee David Weiss, M.D. Chicago: Budlong Press Company, 1978. Part of the "A Doctor Discusses..." series of pamphlets available in many pharmacies, this manual is well illustrated and packed with information on how to talk with children about birth and sex in a warm, natural way.

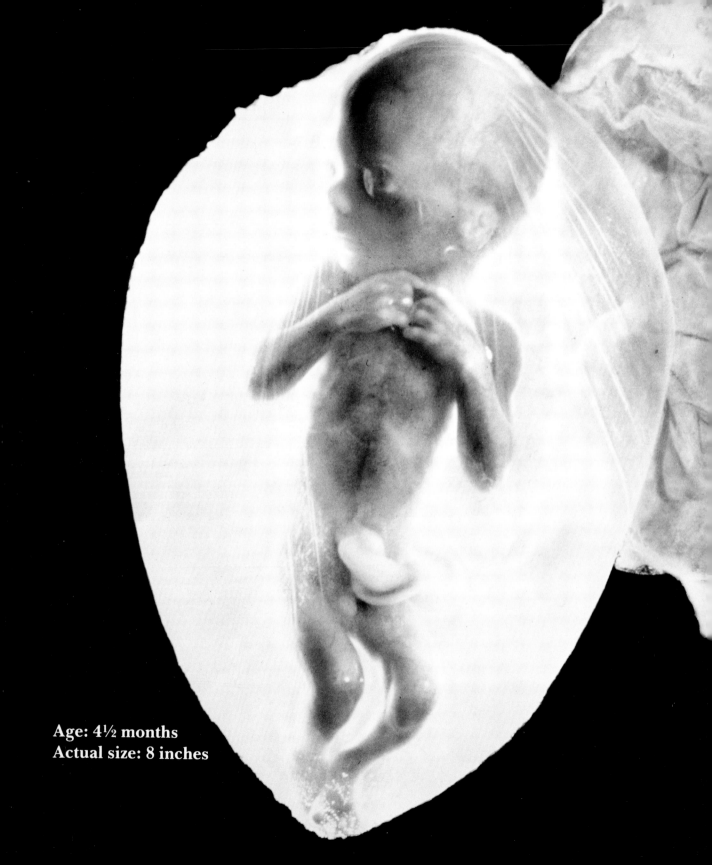

Age: 4½ months
Actual size: 8 inches

Before you were born, you grew in a special place inside your mother's body called her womb, or uterus. There, in a clear sac, you floated in a liquid that was like warm water.

Inside the womb it was dark. You could not see, but you could move, feel, and even hear. You probably heard your parents' voices talking and the sound of your mother's heart beating.

Perhaps you sucked your thumb sometimes, like the unborn baby in the picture.

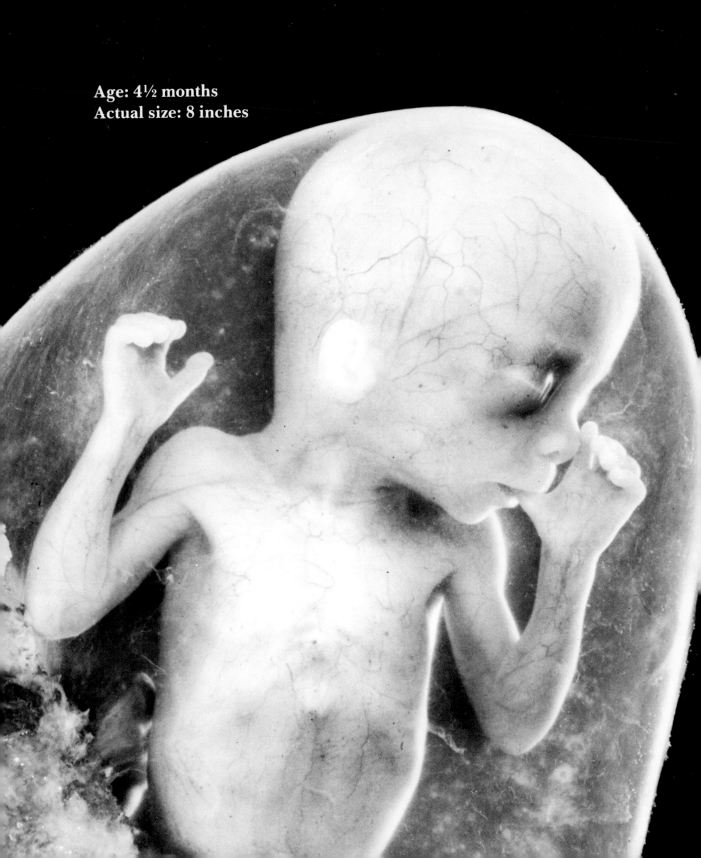

Age: 4½ months
Actual size: 8 inches

When you were born, your body had all the parts you needed to live in the world. But nine months before, when you began, you did not have a head or body, arms or legs, fingers or toes. You started out as one little cell, even smaller than the dot at the end of this sentence.

Half of this cell came from your mother's body, and the other half came from your father's body.

14

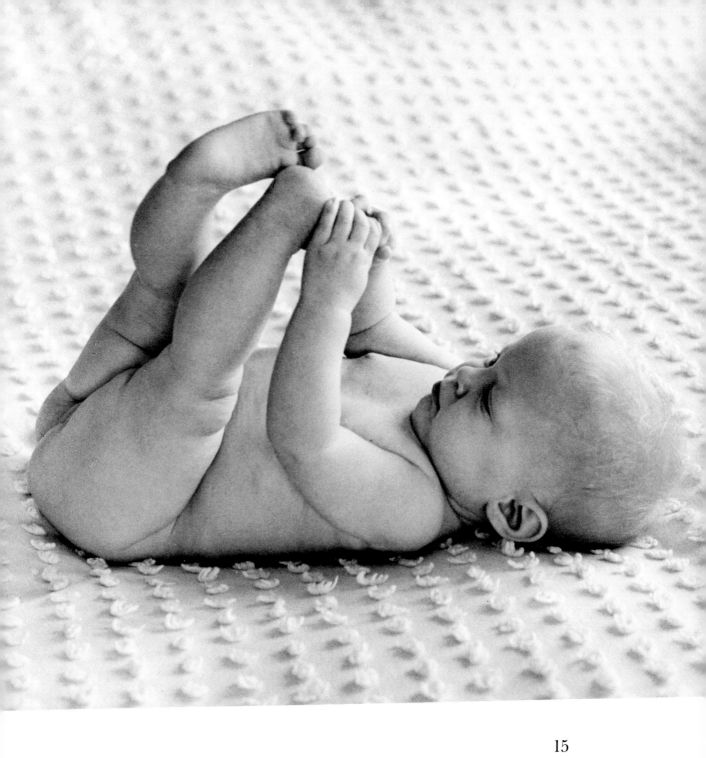

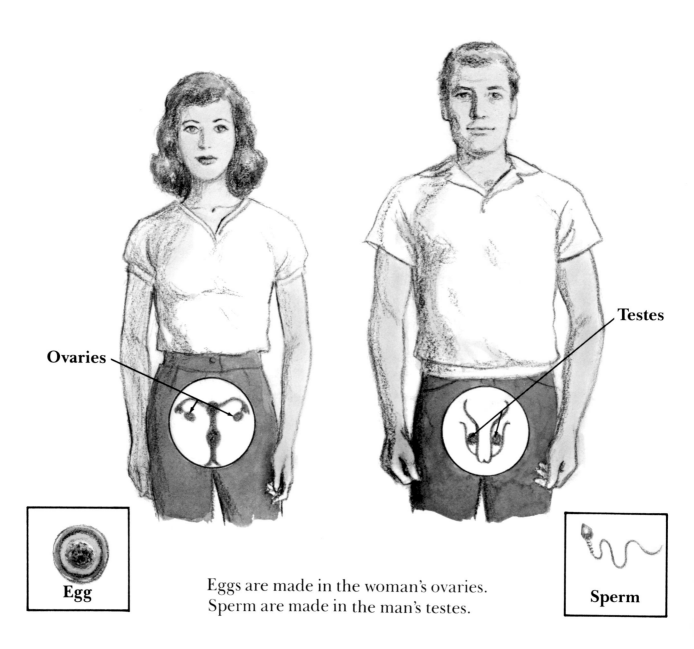

Ovaries

Testes

Egg

Sperm

Eggs are made in the woman's ovaries.
Sperm are made in the man's testes.

16

Inside a woman's body are tiny egg cells.
In a man's body are sperm cells.

The eggs and sperm are so small that we
need a microscope to see them. The egg is
round. It does *not* have a shell like a
chicken's egg. The sperm have long tails
and can swim.

When a sperm and an egg join together,
a special cell is formed. This one cell can
grow into a baby.

All cells shown greatly enlarged.

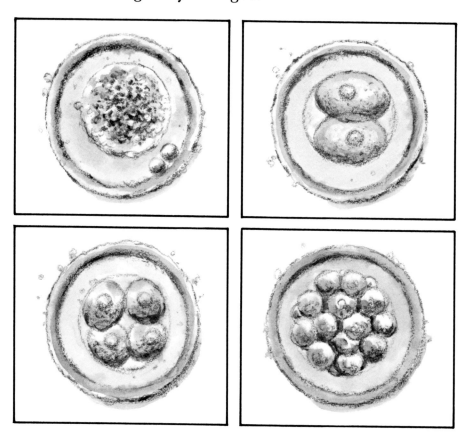

First the special cell divides in half to make two cells. Then each of these cells divides in half again. Now there are four cells. They divide again and again. In a short while, there are hundreds of cells.

After a few weeks of growing, the cells have taken on a shape. It does not look much like a baby, but it is the beginning of one. It will look more and more like a baby as it continues to grow.

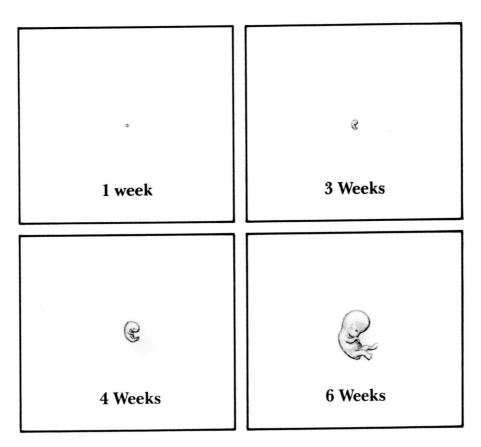

1 week	3 Weeks
4 Weeks	6 Weeks

All above shown actual size.

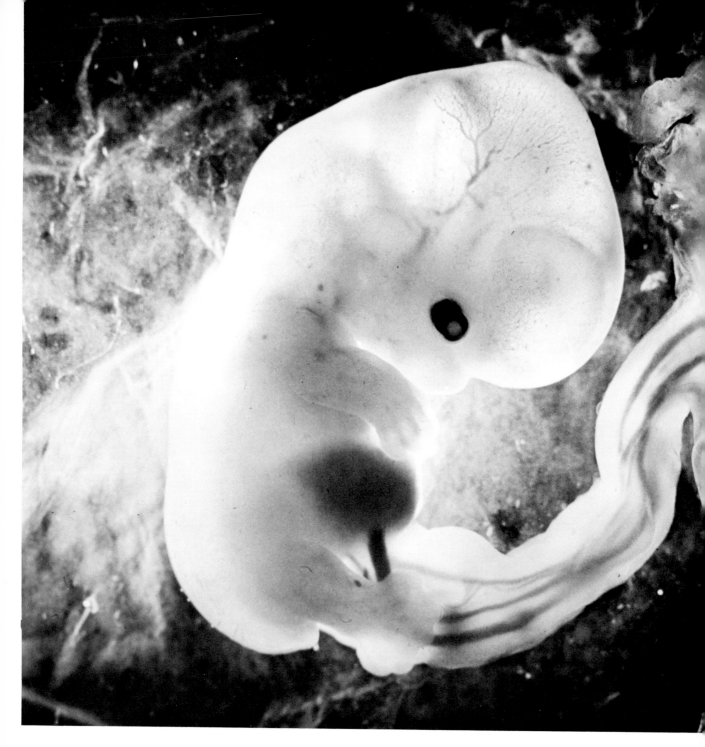

Age: 5½ weeks
Actual size: ⅔ inch

When you had been in your mother's uterus for about six weeks, your hands and feet had started to grow. Your eyes were there, too, and they were wide open because your eyelids had not formed yet.

Inside your body, your heart was already beating!

The photograph here makes the unborn baby seem large, but it is really tiny at this stage: It could fit inside a nutshell.

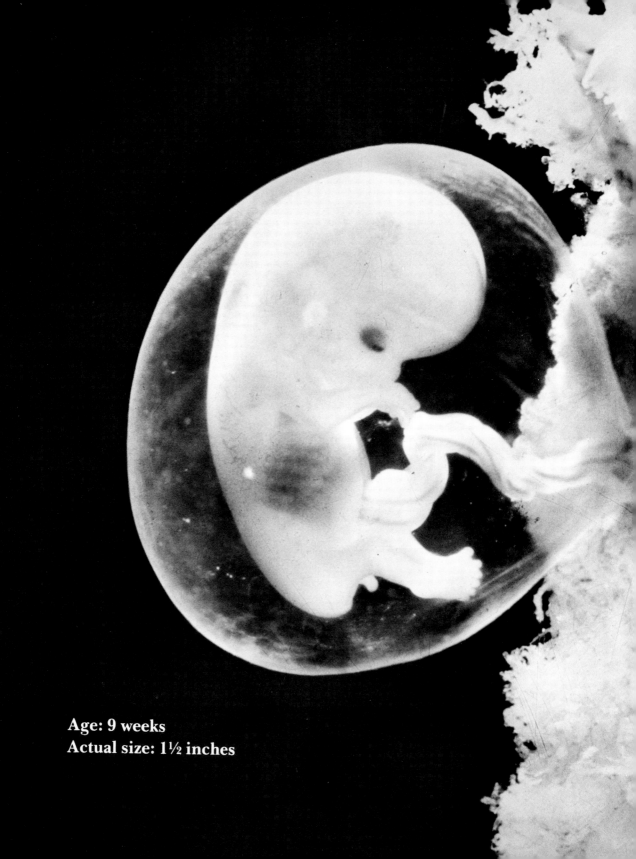

Age: 9 weeks
Actual size: 1½ inches

Already your mother was taking care of you by eating good, nourishing food. Food and oxygen flowed to you from your mother's body through the blood vessels in a tube called the umbilical cord, which was attached to your belly.

Your body wastes were carried away through the blood vessels, too. The umbilical cord worked as a kind of two-way transport system.

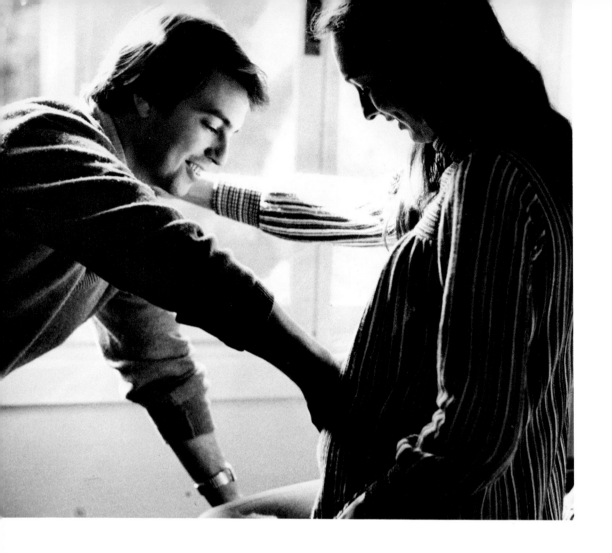

As your muscles grew, you began moving
your arms and legs. Sometimes you turned
a complete somersault in the womb. During
the fourth month, your mother could feel
you moving inside her. Soon others could
feel you moving, too.

24

As the months passed, you grew bigger
and bigger. Your mother's belly had to stretch
way out to make room for you.

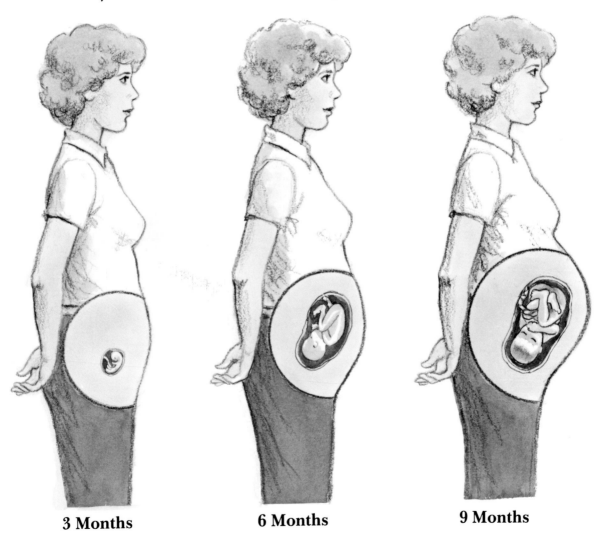

3 Months   **6 Months**   **9 Months**

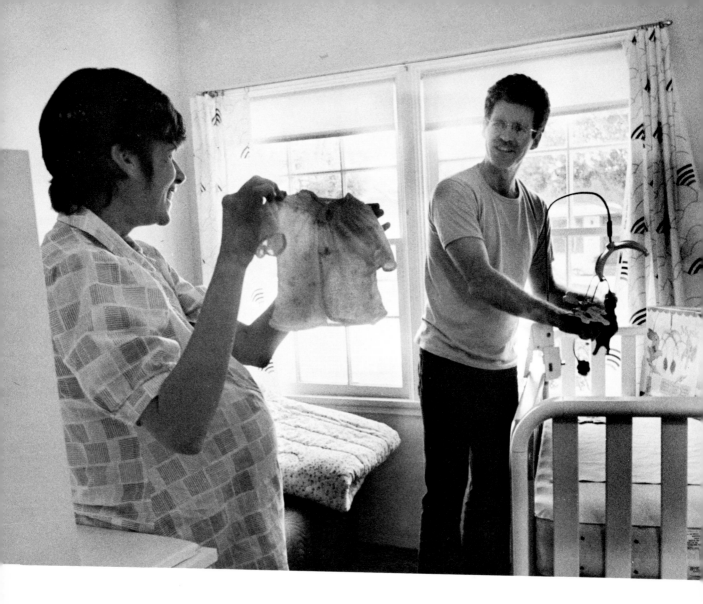

After nine months, you were ready to live
outside the womb. Your mother and father
knew you would be born soon, so they
started getting ready for you.

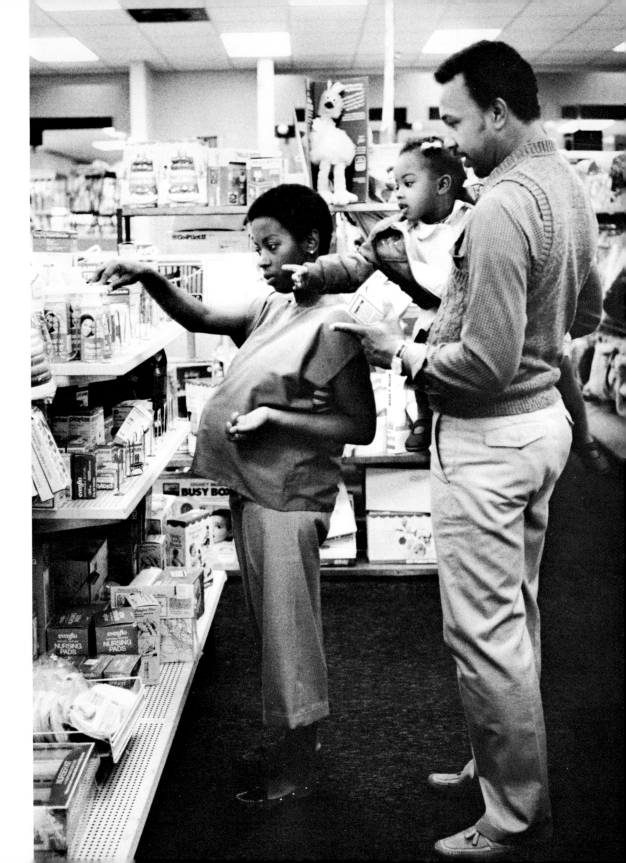

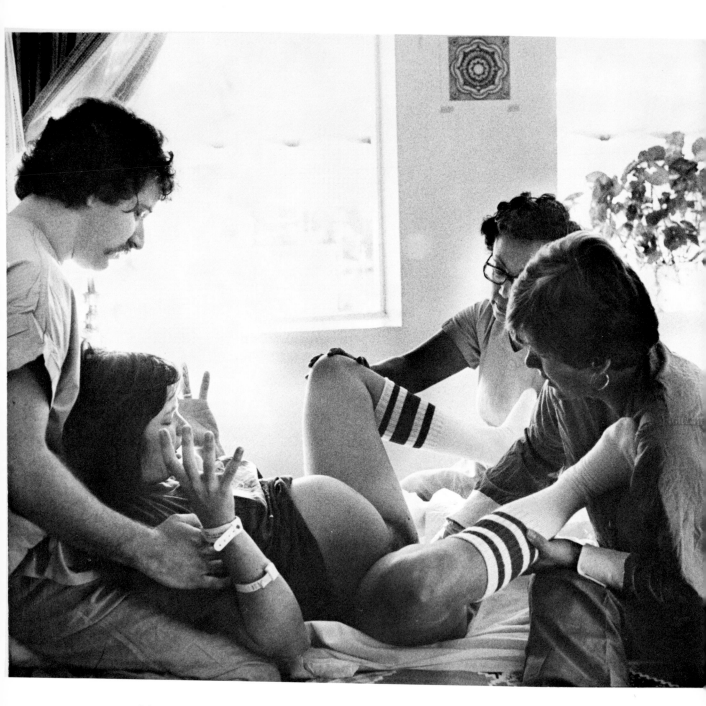

28

One day, your mother felt sharp twinges called labor pains. The uterus was squeezing, or contracting, to push you out through the vagina, a special tunnel leading from the uterus into the world.

When she felt the contractions, your mother knew it was time for the birth. She and your father went to the hospital or childbirth center where you were to be born. Some babies are born at home, and then the doctor or midwife comes to the house.

During labor, your mother had to work hard to push you out. She got help from your father, from nurses, and from her doctor or midwife.

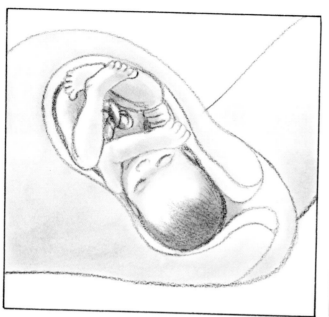 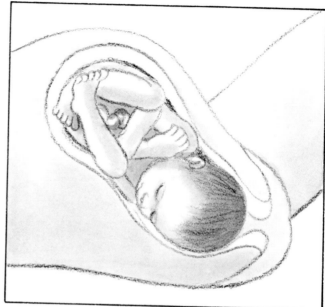

After several hours, the top of your head
appeared. Then your whole body came
through the vagina, which can stretch wide
to let a baby through.

30

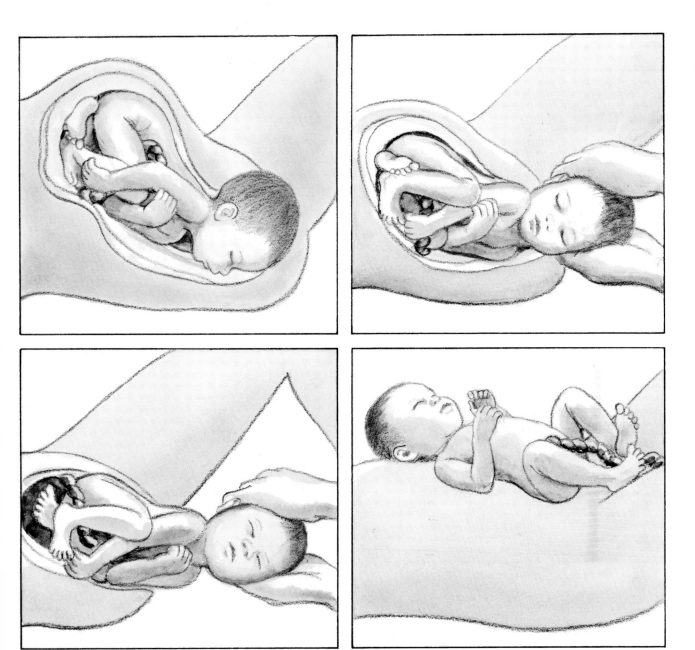

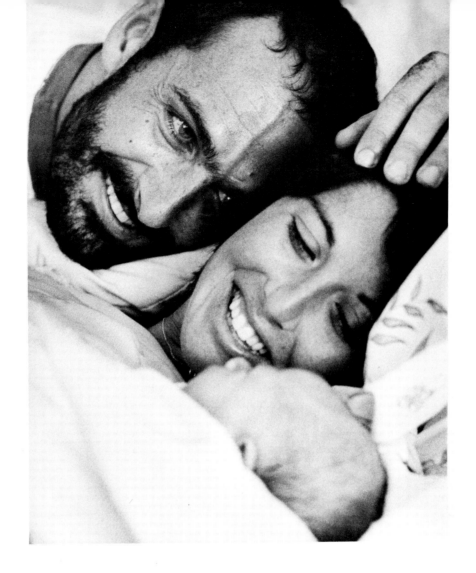

Imagine how excited and happy your parents were when you were finally born!

Now, after months of waiting, they could finally hold you in their arms, getting to know you for the first time.

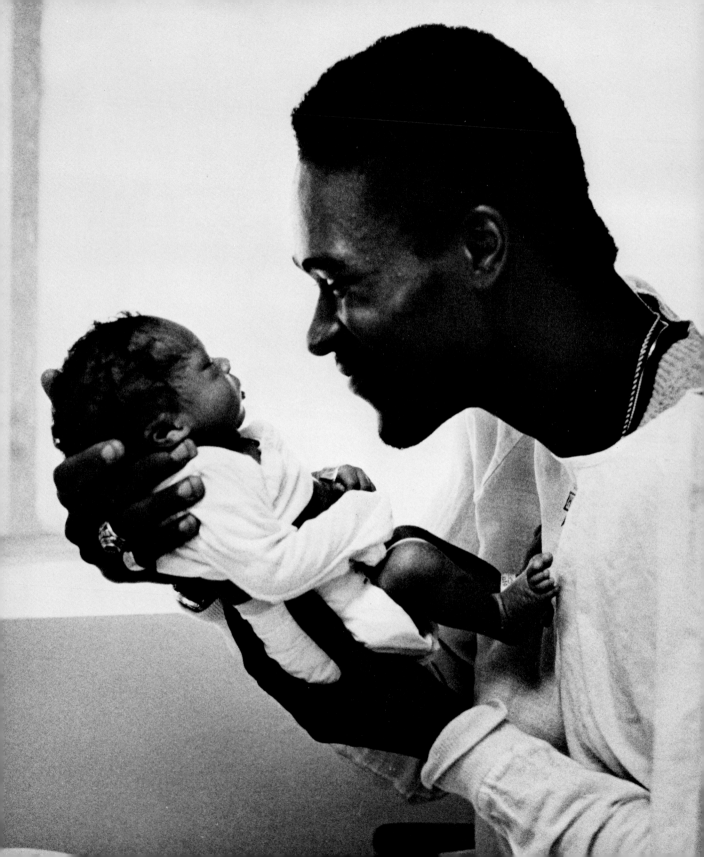

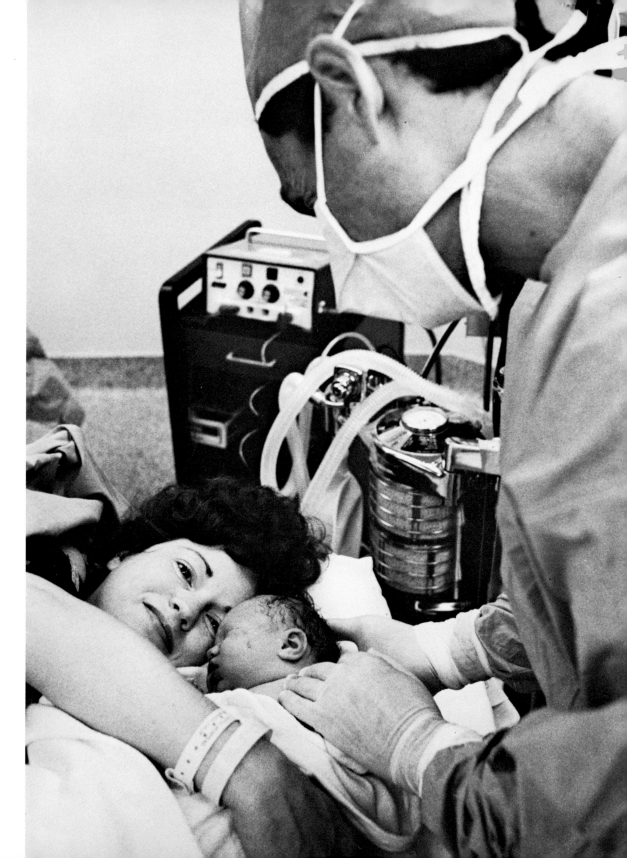

Sometimes a baby cannot be born in the usual way. Perhaps the baby cannot come out easily because of the way it is positioned in the womb. Or maybe the contractions of the uterus are not strong enough to push the baby out.

When this happens, a doctor performs an operation to carefully open the mother's belly and uterus to lift the baby out. The mother is given medication so the operation does not hurt. After the baby is born, the doctor sews up the opening and bandages it so it will heal.

This operation is called a cesarean section.

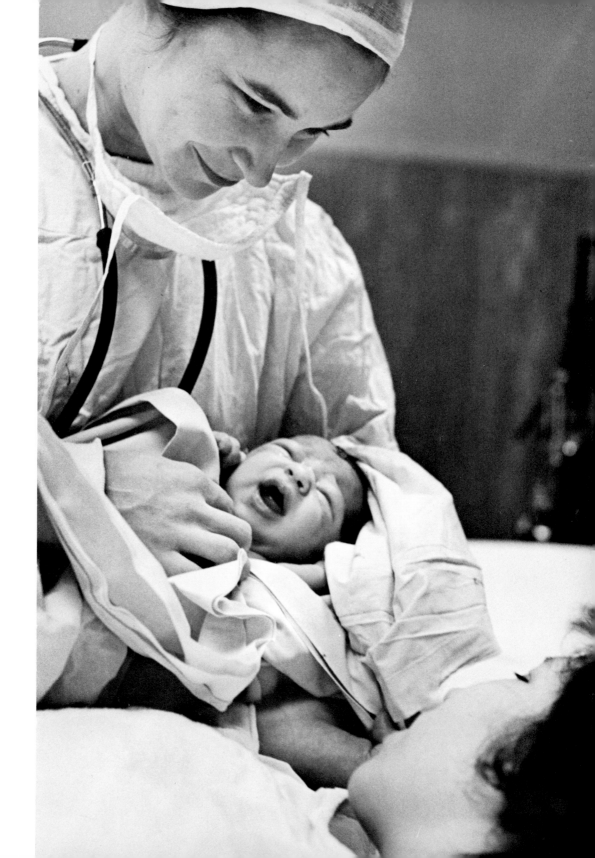

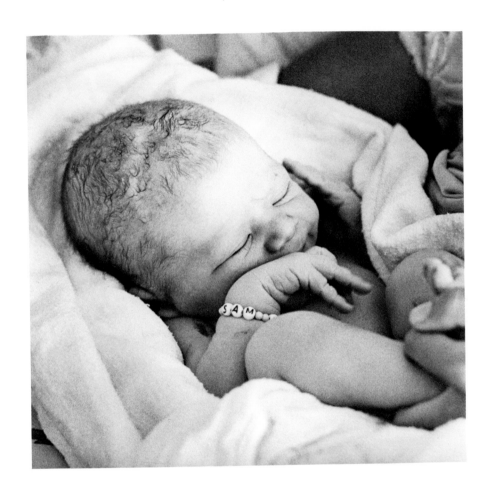

Whichever way you were born, you were
wet and wrinkled. A nurse washed you off
and wrapped you in a warm blanket.

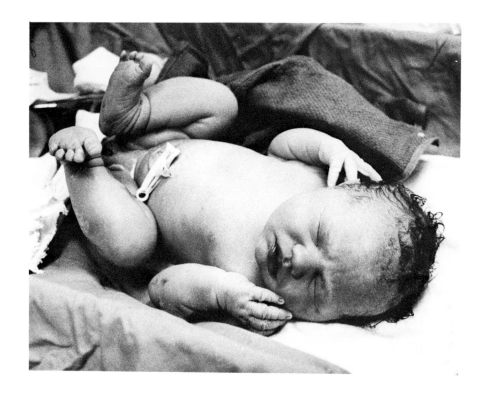

Once you were born, you could eat and breathe on your own. You no longer needed the umbilical cord. The doctor or midwife clamped it shut with a plastic clip and cut it, leaving a piece of the cord attached to your belly. There is no feeling in the cord, so cutting it did not hurt.

In about two weeks, the cord dried up and fell off. Under it was a small, round scab. When that healed, it became your navel, or belly button.

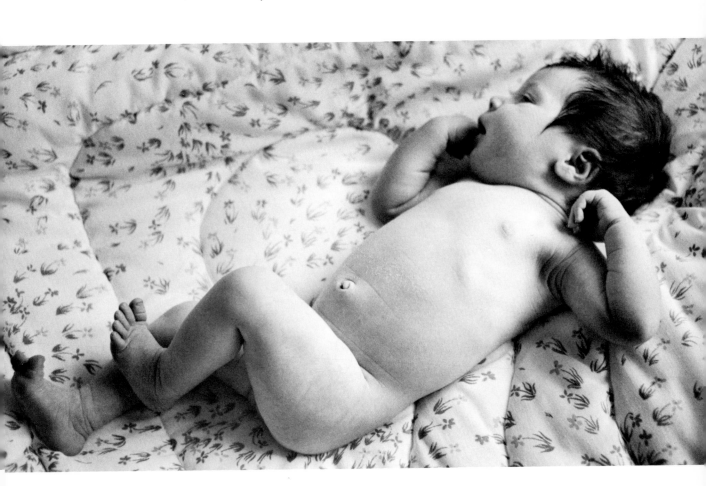

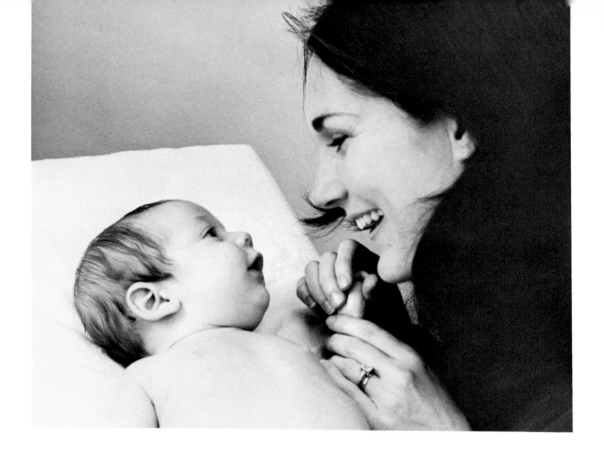

No matter how little and helpless you were, you could see, hear, feel, taste, and smell when you were only a few minutes old. When your parents held you, you could see their faces clearly. When you heard a person's voice, you turned your head toward the sound. If you were crying, you might become quiet when you felt someone holding you.

When you were hungry, you sucked
milk from your mother's breast or a bottle.
And by the time you were a few weeks old,
you learned to tell your mother from other
people simply by your sense of smell.

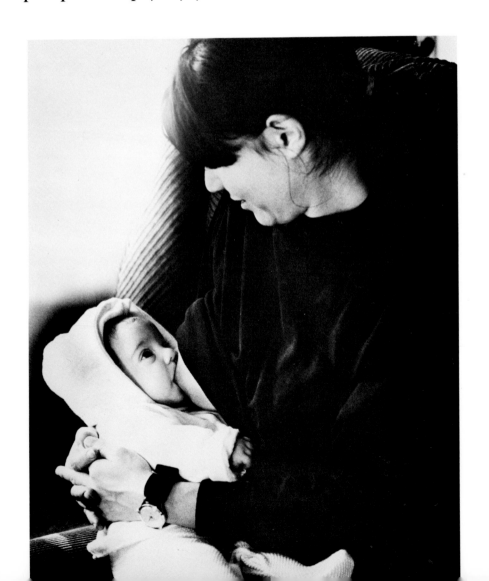

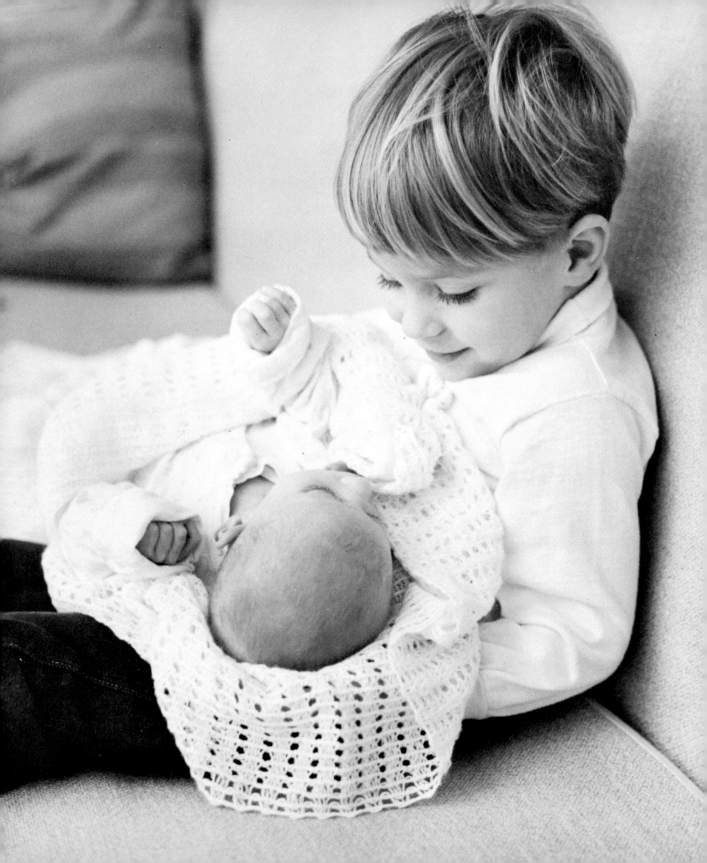

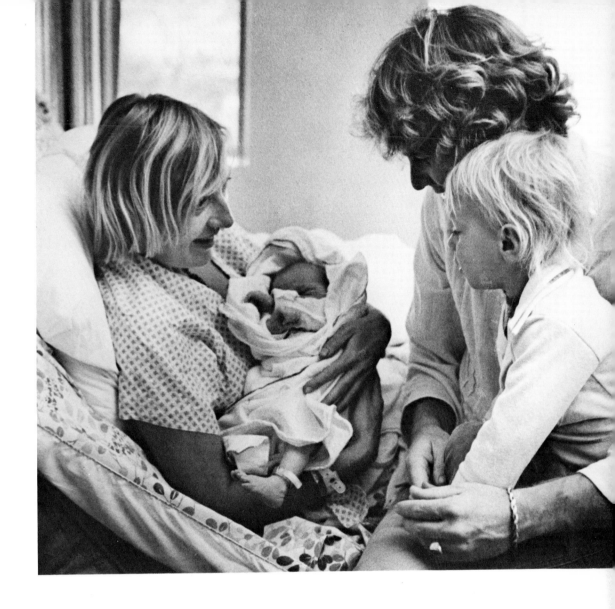

Right from the start, you noticed the
people around you more than anything else.
You were born ready to be part of a family,
ready to learn to love and be loved.

And little by little, you learned more things: to smile and laugh, to play with toys, to crawl and walk, to babble and then say your first words. You were growing up.

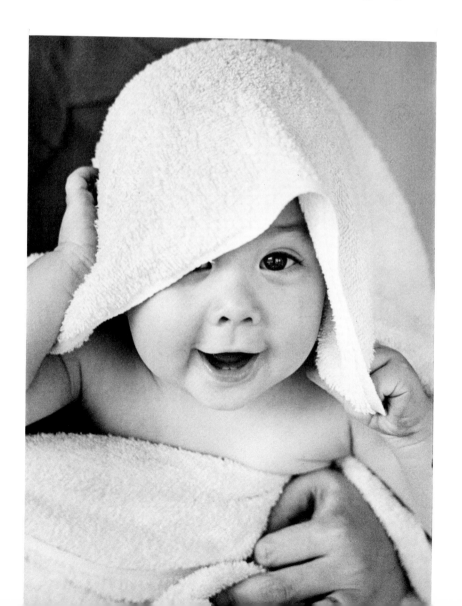

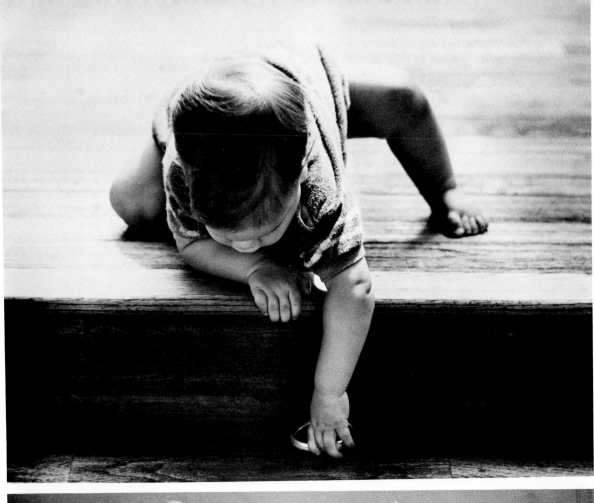

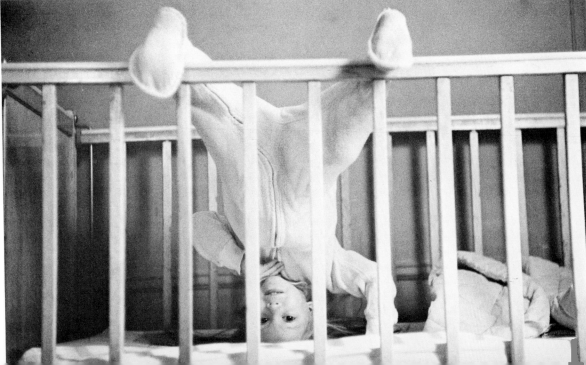

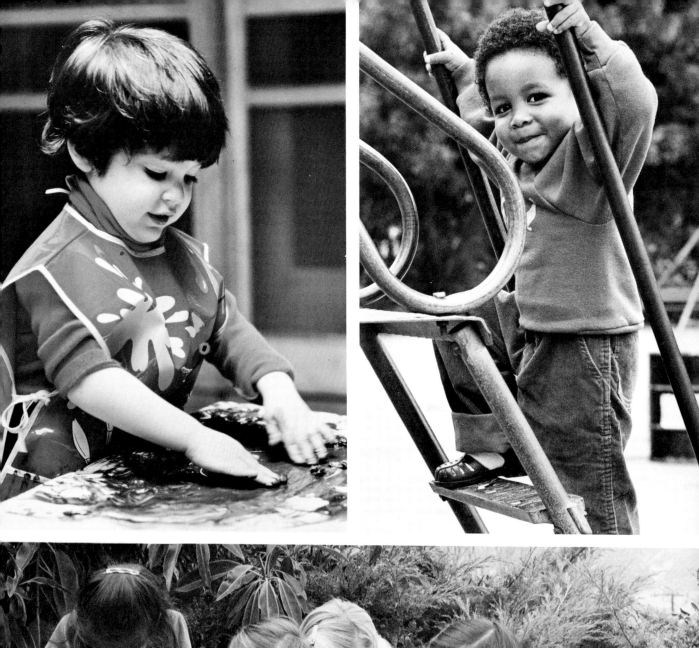
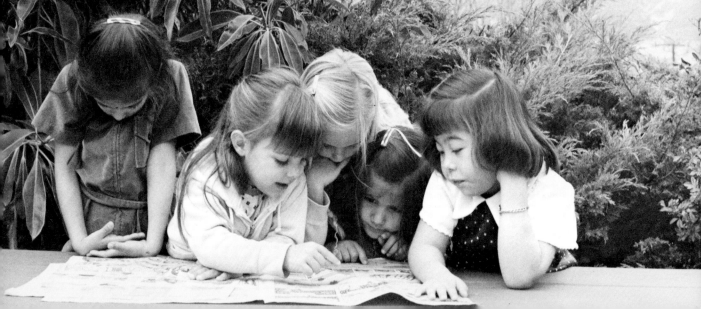

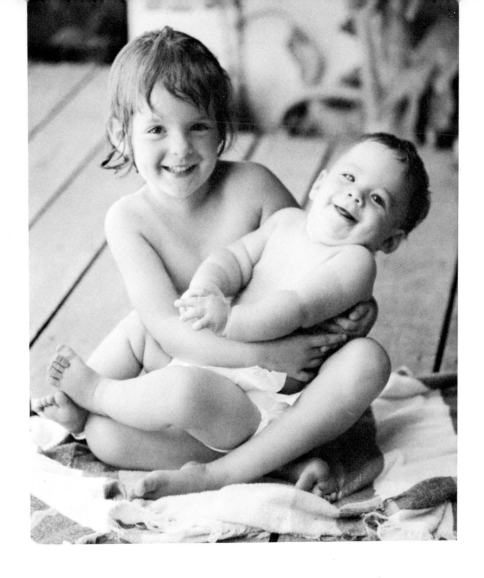

Every newborn baby is the beginning of a person. A person who will one day have feelings and ideas, who will build things, make friends, and have fun. A person who can learn all kinds of new things every day.

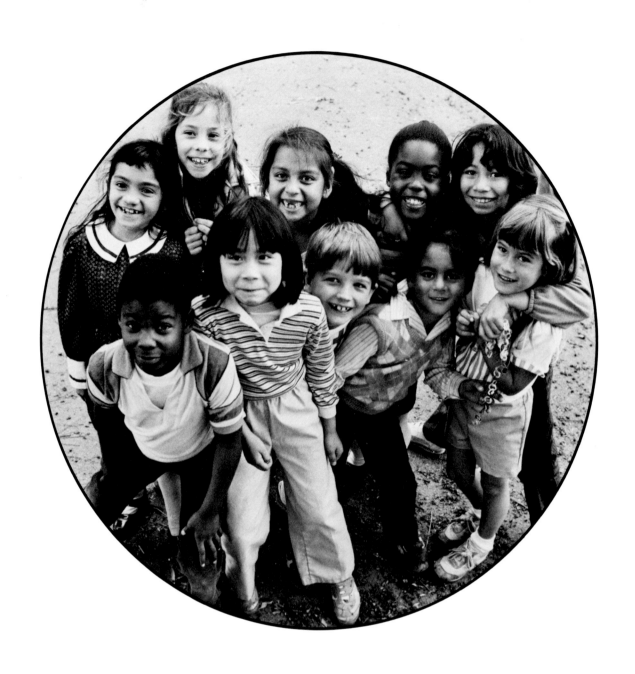

A person just like *you*.